EXERCISE

for
Core Strengthening

edited by
Dr. Irv Rubenstein

VISUAL HEALTH INFORMATION
Tacoma, WA

IMPORTANT INFORMATION:

This book is intended to be used as a reference book by qualified medical or fitness professionals. Thus, anyone using the exercises listed in this book without appropriate training in the field of fitness and exercise, or without the prior consent of a physician or therapeutic professional, may be placing themselves at risk for an injury. The exercises are provided as options, *not prescriptions*, and are therefore to be used in concert with an experienced professional's education and guidelines. VHI is not responsible or liable, directly or indirectly, for any damages whatsoever resulting in injury from the information contained in this work.

Cover design by Roxanne Carrington
Publication design and layout by Bethany Maines
Illustrations from the libraries of VHI

10 9 8 7 6 5 4 3 2 1

Printed in the United States of America

Publisher's Cataloging-in-Publication
(Provided by Quality Books, Inc.)

Exercise ideas for core strengthening / edited by Irv Rubenstein.
    p. cm.
    ISBN 1–929343–06–X

    1. Back exercises.   I. Rubenstein, Irv.

GV508.E944 2005   613.7'1
                      QB105–200075

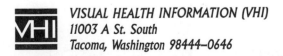

VISUAL HEALTH INFORMATION (VHI)
11003 A St. South
Tacoma, Washington 98444–0646

Book Orders: 1–800–356–0709
All Other Inquiries: 1–253–536–4922

CONTENTS

Introduction

The material in this collection is designed to meet the needs of medical and fitness professionals who work with the strength needs of patients and clients. It is a compilation of exercise ideas and options for strengthening and conditioning the core.

This work brings together the creativity of many experts in fitness and rehabilitation who have designed "kits" for Visual Health Information (Tacoma, WA). It is not the purpose or intent of this collection to represent each and every possible exercise option for each part of the body. Nor is it the intent to describe and define when and how to use or not use any one exercise for any particular client or athlete, especially where a therapeutic consideration is warranted. Rather, it is designed simply as a resource, a reference for those who help others get in shape, to improve function or form.

Therapists and trainers often have limited resources — either working with a minimum of gym equipment or in people's homes. Creativity becomes all the more important under these circumstances. When a client's unique needs or interests confront a therapist or trainer, his understanding of biomechanics and anatomy may be challenged in ways that require him to search for options. This collection was designed and should be used to find ways to get the same results with a variety of methods.

What is "Core Strength"?

Core strength is a relatively new phrase in the fitness field. In the past, core strength referred to exercises that were considered fundamental in the conditioning of athletes. Exercises such as the squat, bench press, dead lift, clean, hang clean, etc. were regarded as absolutely essential, i.e. core, in the training of strength and power athletes.

In the mid-1990s, researchers in Australia elucidated the role of some of the intrinsic muscles of the trunk in stabilizing the spine. In particular, the transverse abdominis (TVA) of the abdominal area and the multifidi and rotatores of the low back were found to be absolutely essential in the proper function and control of the lumbar spine. "Core" then took on the meaning of torso or trunk stabilizers.

In the past, abdominal strengthening was considered the solution to low back problems or weakness. In the 1950s, Drs. Hans Krause and P. Williams developed a conditioning program for the abdominals which they stated would resolve or prevent most low back problems.

Then, in the 1980s, New Zealand physiotherapist, Robin McKenzie, developed a sequence of exercises for the lumbar spine and stabilizing assistors (pelvic muscles) that put more emphasis on the posterior trunk muscles.

Today the fitness field incorporates all those ideas plus some from a variety of protocols such as yoga, Pilates, foam rollers, stability balls, etc. into an combination of abdominal and low back exercises that we call "core exercises". There are several definitions of the "core" but for the purposes of this book, **Exercise Ideas for Core Strength,** we define core as the muscles of the lower torso that stabilize and move the lumbar spine, in its relation to the pelvis. We include the pelvis because it is the base of the spine. Controlling its movements supports and controls the lumbar spine movements. However, we do not intend to cover all the exercise options for the hips, which are technically pelvic exercises, too. In our Exercise Ideas series, Exercise Ideas for the Lower Body addresses the hip-moving muscles. This book addresses the musculature of the pelvis that directly relate to those of the lower torso.

Dividing this area of the body into simple chapter-like sections is not easy due to the inter-relatedness of the various muscles of the core. Rather than try to lay out a progression, which is somewhat subjective and variable according to a person's needs and abilities, we have chosen group the exercises into four core training concepts: Core Control, Core Stability, Core Strength, and Core Function. Each chapter is subdivided into Anterior and Posterior sections. The anterior section addresses the abdominal wall; the posterior section addresses the lumbar region. Each section includes some pelvic muscle exercises.

For some of the exercises, it will be evident that the crossover activation of anterior and posterior muscles belies the idea of isolation. For example, the TVA is a major stabilizing component of any activities involving the lumbar spine, even the appendages, and is part of the anterior portion of the core, isolating it out of the section on posterior muscles is impossible.

Core control refers to exercises that are relatively isometric in that little to no movement of the lumbar spine or pelvis should or does occur.

Core stability refers to exercises that require multi-directional control of the lumbar spine, usually with some component of instability. This may come from an exercise tool, such as a therapeutic ball, or from something as simple as single dumbbell held in one hand.

Core strength exercises are those that engage large groups of, or large actions by, the muscles of the anterior or posterior walls. They are less subtle in nature, involving forceful contractions of the prime movers in a particular direction.

Core function refers to exercises that involve anterior and posterior muscles working together, often with pelvic muscles, to make movements in positions that duplicate movements of daily living or a sport.

Exercise Ideas for Core Strength provides the trainer with over 180 exercises for the muscles and joints of the lower torso and pelvis. It is not meant to be a therapeutic guide although many of the exercises are potentially therapeutic. The exercises in each section will be ordered in a reasonable manner from easiest to hardest. This distinction is not black and white. Therefore, the reader will have to be lenient with our system as well as diligent in his or her application of these exercise ideas.

Finally, as in any book of this nature, a disclaimer is necessary. Thus, anyone using the exercises listed in this book without appropriate training in the field of fitness and exercise, or without the prior consent of a physician or therapeutic professional, may be placing his/her clients or him / herself at risk for an injury. The exercises are provided as options, not prescriptions, and are therefore to be used in concert with an experienced professional's education and guidelines.

Chapter 1: Core Control

A person is said to have core control when the lower abdominal, low back, and pelvic muscles work together to lock in the lumbar spine in order to protect it from errant motions and secure a firm base upon which all movements of the extremities can occur. For the sake of simplicity, this core control section refers to exercises that are relatively isometric in that little to no movement of the lumbar spine or pelvis occurs. Thus, the anterior muscles — the abdominals and/or hip flexors — lock in against any forces that are trying to extend the spine; and the posterior muscles — the erector spinae and the intrinsic muscles of the lumbar spine — lock in against any flexion moments. Finally, pelvic muscles — the gluteals and the hip flexors and, undetectably, the pelvic floor muscles — stabilize the pelvis to prevent rotation or tilt. Most core control exercises are progressed by increasing the duration of a holding position, then increasing repetitions. Load or intensity is not as instrumental in making control improvements.

Anterior — 51 exercises

Posterior — 21 exercises

Isometric Abdominal

Lying on back with knees bent, tighten stomach by pressing elbows down. Hold.

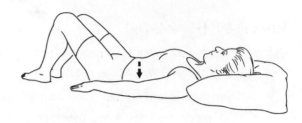

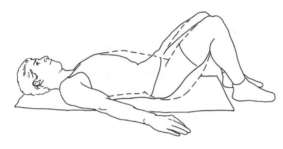

Pelvic Tilt

Lie on back, legs bent. Exhale, tilting top of pelvis back, pubic bone up, to flatten lower back. Inhale, rolling pelvis opposite way, top forward, pubic bone down, arch in back.

Extremity Flexion (Hook-Lying)

Tighten stomach and slowly lower right arm over head until back begins to arch. Hold. Return slowly, keeping trunk rigid.

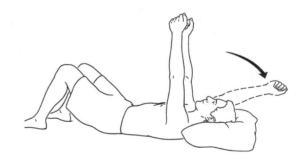

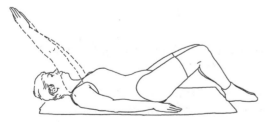

Rib Cage Arms

Lie on back, legs bent, arms by sides. Inhale, lifting arms over head. Exhale, returning.

NOTE: Avoid lifting rib cage and abdomen.

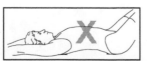

Bent Leg Lift (Hook-Lying)

Tighten stomach and slowly raise one leg from floor. Hold. Return slowly, keeping trunk rigid.

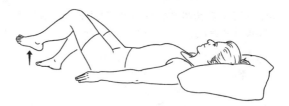

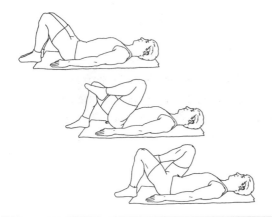

Knee Fold

Lie on back, legs bent, arms by sides. Exhale, lifting knee to chest. Inhale, returning. Keep abdominals flat, navel to spine.

Combination (Hook-Lying)

Tighten stomach and slowly raise one leg and lower opposite arm over head. Hold. Return slowly, keeping trunk rigid.

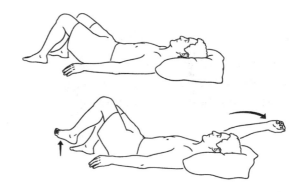

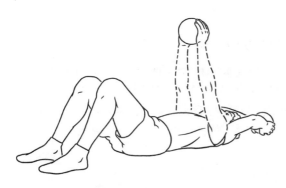

Cranial Flexion: Over Head Arm Extension (Medicine Ball)

Lie with knees bent, arms beyond head, holding a ball. Pull ball up to above face.

Diagonal Over Head Arm Extension: Supine (Medicine Ball)

Lie with knees bent, arms back above right shoulder, holding ball. Pull ball across to opposite hip.

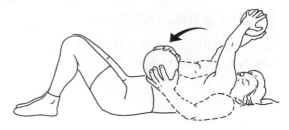

Heel Walk (Hook-Lying)

Tighten stomach and slowly walk feet forward in short steps until legs are nearly straight, or until back begins to arch.

Unilateral Isometric Hip Flexion

Tighten stomach muscles and raise knee to outstretched arm. Push gently, keeping arm straight, trunk rigid. Hold.

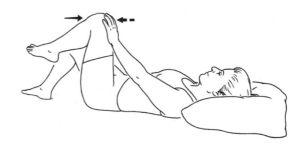

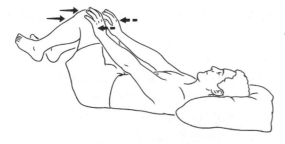

Bilateral Isometric Hip Flexion

Tighten stomach muscles and raise both knees to outstretched arms. Push gently, keeping arms straight, trunk rigid. Hold.

Straight Leg Raise

Tighten stomach muscles and slowly raise locked leg from floor. Hold.

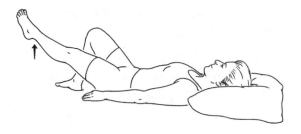

Straight Leg Raise, Advanced

With knees bent and feet away from floor, slowly straighten leg, keeping stomach tight. Hold.

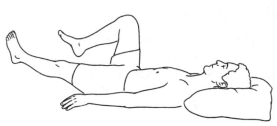

Single Leg Circle

Lie on back, one leg bent, other leg straight up. Inhale, circling leg across body, and exhale while circling down and around to beginning. Maintain still pelvis; avoid rocking. Keep circle small.

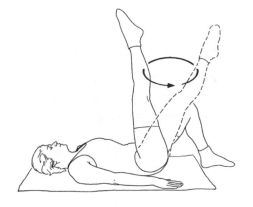

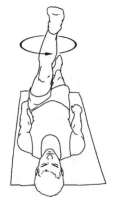

Single Leg Circle (Intermediate / Advanced)

Lie on back, leg extended on mat, other leg straight up. Inhale, circling leg across body, and exhale as you finish circling down and around to beginning. Maintain still pelvis; avoid rocking. Keep circle small.

Scissor

Lie on back, legs straight up, hands under lower hips. Exhale, splitting legs with a pulse. Inhale, changing legs. Keep hips flat. Do not let bottom leg go below 45°.

NOTE: Keep navel to spine, back flat.

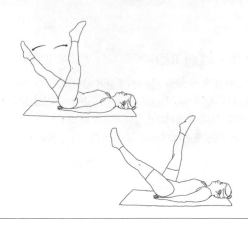

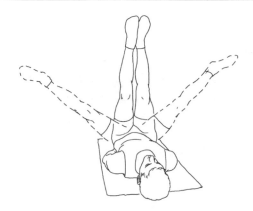

Straight Leg Open / Close

Lie on back, legs straight up, hands under lower hips, head down. Inhale, opening legs to side. Exhale, closing legs.

NOTE: Keep navel to spine, back flat.

Lower Lift

Lie on back, legs straight up, slightly turned out, hands under hips. Exhale, slowly lowering legs a few degrees. Inhale, returning. Press heels together. Knees may be slightly bent, leaving quads released.

NOTE: Keep navel to spine, back flat.

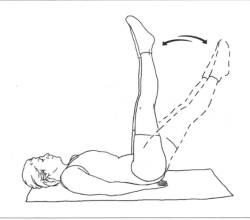

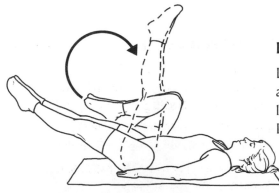

Double Bicycle

Lie on back, legs bent and together. In a continuous motion, exhale, extending legs out to 45°, then toward ceiling. Inhale, bending legs to return.

Lower Lift (Intermediate / Advanced)

Lie on back, legs straight up, slightly turned out, heels touching. Hands behind head, lift head and upper torso. Exhale, lowering legs to 45°. Inhale, returning. Keep head and torso up, low back flat.

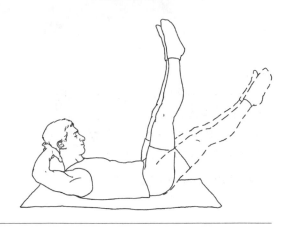

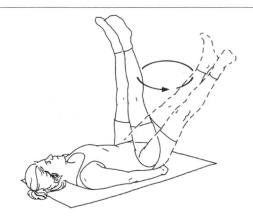

Corkscrew

Lie on back, legs straight up, slightly turned out, heels touching, hands under lower hips. Inhale, reaching legs out to one side. Exhale, circling with legs. Maintain legs above 45°. Avoid arching spine off mat.

Frog

Lie on back, legs bent in, slightly turn out, heels touching. Exhale, extending legs out to 45°, keeping heels touching. Inhale, bringing knees back in.

NOTE: Beginners keep feet parallel.

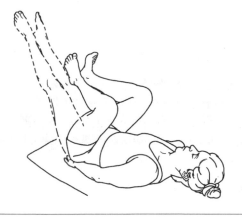

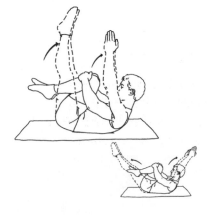

Double Leg Stretch

Lie on back, hands holding knees to chest. Exhale, curling up head and upper torso to knees. Holding curl, inhale and extend arms and legs toward ceiling. Exhale, bringing legs and arms back in.

NOTE: Keep navel to spine, back flat. Progress to extending arms and legs to 45°.

Toe Touch

Lie on back, legs folded to chest, arms by sides. Exhale, lowering leg to just touch toes to mat. Inhale, returning knee to chest. Keep abdominals flat, navel to spine.

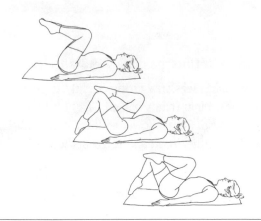

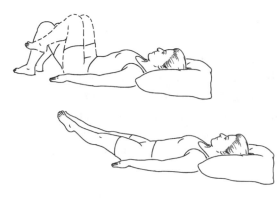

Double Knee Lift

With knees bent, slowly bring both knees toward chest, keeping stomach tight. Then extend legs without touching feet to floor. Hold. Return slowly, keeping trunk rigid.

Open Leg Balance

Sit straight, hands under thighs, legs hip width apart. Press navel to spine and lean back to balance on seat, legs bent in air. Exhale, extending legs straight, grasping ankles. Hold.

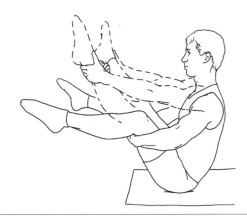

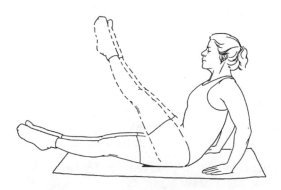

Hip / Leg Raise

Leaning back on hands. Exhale, raising legs toward ceiling. Inhale, lowering to just off mat. Keep torso still and arms bent slightly.

Side Leg Beat

Lie on side, back straight along edge of mat, legs 30° in front of torso. Turned out slightly, raise legs a few inches. Beat heels together lightly, inhaling and exhaling.

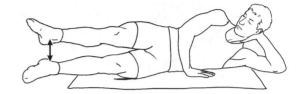

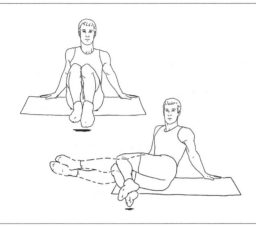

Can-Can

Leaning back on hands, bend legs 90° and raise slightly off floor. Exhale, twisting hips to side, and extend legs straight. Inhale, bending legs and returning.

Side Lower Lift

Sit balanced on side of hip, supported on forearm in front, hand in back. Legs slightly turned out, raise a few inches from mat. Exhale, lifting legs. Inhale, lowering to slightly off mat.

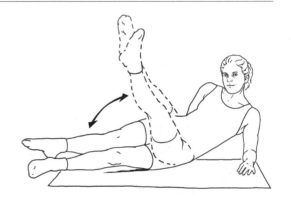

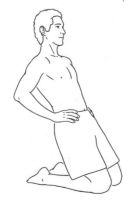

Backward Lean (Kneeling)

Slowly lean backward, keeping stomach tight, trunk rigid. Hold.

On Target: Finding Spine Stability

Lie on roller, feet on floor. Arch and flatten entire spine. Think of tacking spine to roller, then letting go. Continue with less and less motion. Come to rest. Be aware of muscles being used. This is the target position for many supine exercises.

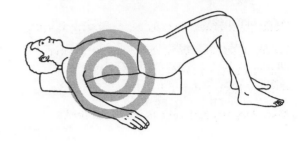

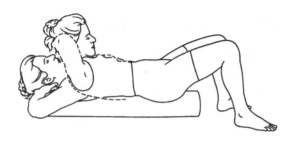

Abdominal: Strengthening

Lie on roller, knees bent, feet on floor, hands behind head. Keeping lower body on roller, abdomen taut, curl head and shoulders up. Exhale during curl, inhale on return. Hold.

Abdominal: Strengthening Varied Arm Positions

1. Cross protected
2. At sides supported
3. Outstretched
4. One arm outstretched
5. Behind head
6. One arm behind head

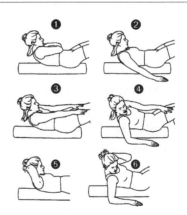

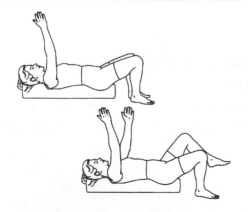

Stabilization Routine

Lie on roller. Holding trunk still, lift limbs in various combinations. Hold each position.

Dead Bug: Lower Abdominal Strengthening

Lie on roller, legs in air. Bend and straighten legs at a level to maintain abdominal tension. Keep trunk still. Hold.

Note: Bring legs back close to body when tired.

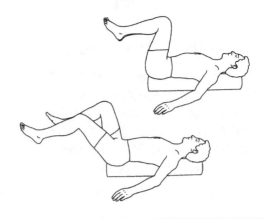

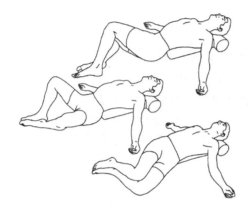

Lower Trunk Rotation / Pelvic Opening

Lean on roller, spine rotated, knees together on one side. Open legs as far as possible. Rotate to other side. Hold each position.

Hip Hiking

Lie with horizontal roller supporting back, short full rollers under ankles. Hips off floor and straight, shorten one side of body and lengthen the other as legs roll back and forth. Hold each position.

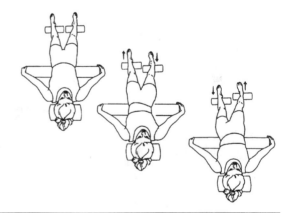

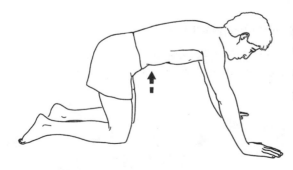

Stabilization: Abdominus Contraction Quadruped

On all fours, tighten stomach, pulling navel toward spine. Keep hips, pelvis, and spine still.

Cat / Camel: Flexion / Extension

Knees and hands on rollers:

1. Cat: Buttocks up, arch spine segmentally, bottom to top: lift chest as head moves backward, look up.
2. Camel: Reverse movement. Close eyes, lower head, tuck chin, compress chest and abdomen, round back. Hold.

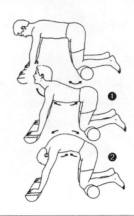

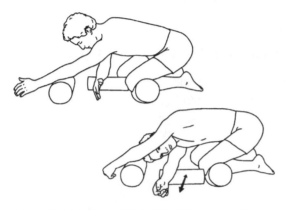

Cross Trunk Rotation

Crouch on roller, straight arm on full roller, smaller, full roller in cross position under bent arm. Slide bent arm across body, twisting trunk, stretching back of shoulder. Lean on moving arm. Elongate trunk with straight arm. Hold.

Pelvic Tilt

Gently rotate pelvis forward and backward.

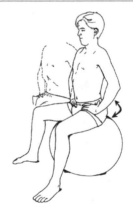

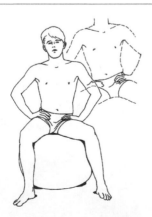

Lateral Pelvic Tilt

Gently move hips from side to side.

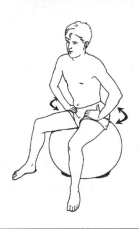

Pelvic Circles

Gently rotate pelvis in clockwise then counterclockwise circles.

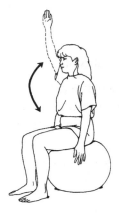

Alternating Arm Raise: Sitting

Raise one arm above head and return. Repeat with other arm.

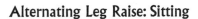

Alternating Leg Raise: Sitting

Raise bent knee and return. Repeat with other leg.

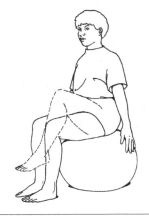

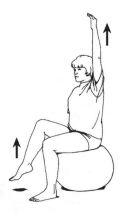

Opposite Arm and Leg Raise: Sitting

Raise opposite leg and arm and return. Repeat with other limbs.

Same Side Arm and Leg Raise: Sitting

Raise same side arm and leg and
return. Repeat with opposite side.

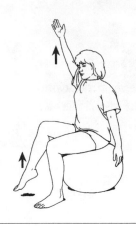

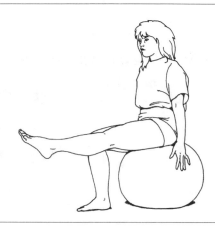

Leg Extension: Sitting

Straighten knee and return.
Repeat with opposite side.

Jumping Jack (Aquatic)

Jump, moving both legs apart, while lifting
arms out from sides. Jump again, bringing
legs together and arms back to start.

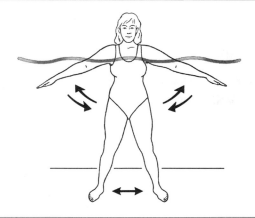

Isometric Gluteals

Tighten buttock muscles. Hold.

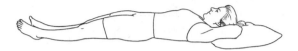

Pelvic Tilt: Anterior – Legs Straight (Supine)

Rotate pelvis up and arch back. Hold. Relax.

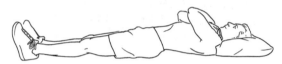

Gluteal Sets

Tighten buttocks while pressing pelvis to floor. Hold.

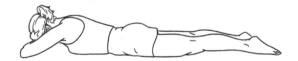

Neck / Back Isometric (Prone)

With pelvis slightly tilted, tense the muscles of back and neck without moving or lifting trunk. Hold.

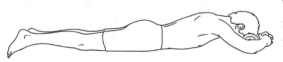

Bent Knee Lift (Prone)

Abdomen and head supported,
bend one knee and slowly raise hip.
Avoid arching low back. Hold.

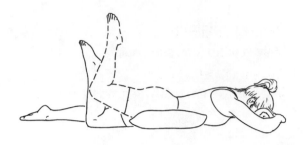

Straight Leg Raise (Prone)

Abdomen and head supported, keep
one knee locked and raise leg at hip.
Avoid arching low back. Hold.

Hip Extension (Prone)

Lift one leg from floor, keeping
knee locked. Hold.

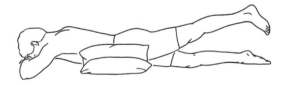

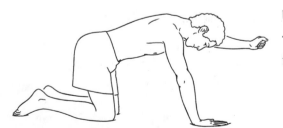

Upper Extremity Extension (All Fours)

Tighten stomach and raise one arm parallel to
floor. Hold. Return slowly, keeping trunk rigid.

Upper / Lower Extremity Extension (All Fours)

Tighten stomach and raise one leg and opposite arm. Hold. Return slowly, keeping trunk rigid.

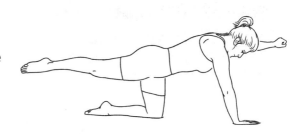

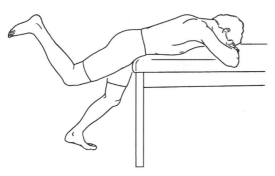

Hip Extension: Unilateral – Support

Leaning torso on table, lift leg, knee bent. Hold. Repeat with other leg.

Hip Extension: Bilateral – Support

Holding onto table, raise both legs from floor knees bent. Hold.

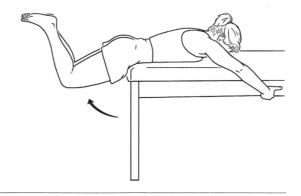

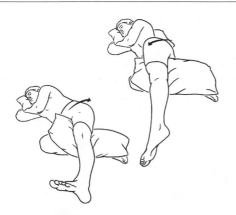

Lumbar Rotation (Side-Lying)

Lying on side, gently rotate hips back and forth, keeping trunk straight. Put pillow between knees to support pelvis.

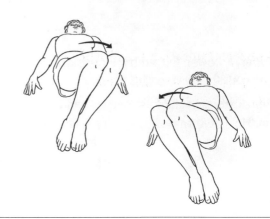

Lumbar Rotation (Non-Weight Bearing)

Feet on floor, slowly rock knees from side to side in small, pain-free range of motion. Allow lower back to rotate slightly.

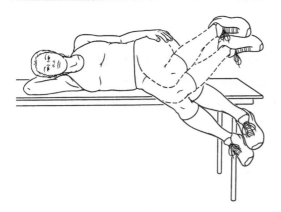

Lumbar Side-Bend: Legs Over Edge (Side-Lying)

Lying on side, knees bent, lower legs over edge of table, rotate legs up at knees.

Hip Hinge: Double Leg (Gymball)

From sitting, roll out so ball supports shoulder blades, back straight, knees over ankles. Lower and raise hips, keeping back straight.

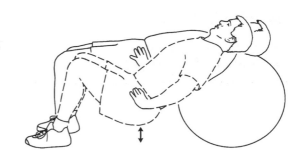

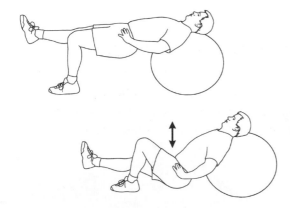

Hip Hinge: Single Leg (Gymball)

From sitting, roll out so ball supports shoulder blades, back straight. Straighten one leg. Other leg bent, knee over ankle, lower and raise hips. Repeat with other leg.

Bridging: Double Leg (Gymball)

Lie on back, calves on ball. Slowly raise and lower buttocks.

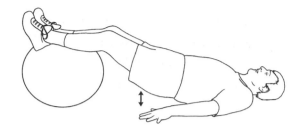

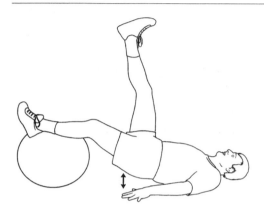

Bridging: Single Leg (Gymball)

Lie on back, calves on ball. With one leg vertical, slowly raise and lower buttocks. Repeat with other leg up.

Hamstring Curl: Double Leg (Gymball)

Lie on back, calves on ball, buttocks on floor. Raise buttocks then roll ball toward buttocks. Hold, or lower buttocks to floor, between rolls.

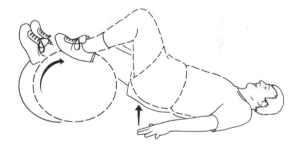

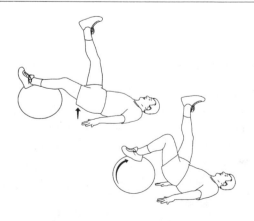

Hamstring Curl: Single Leg (Gymball)

Lie on back, calves on ball. Raise buttocks and hold. With one leg vertical, roll ball toward buttocks. Hold, or lower buttocks to floor, between rolls. Repeat with other leg up.

Strengthening: Hip Extension – Resisted

With tubing around one ankle, face
anchor and pull leg straight back.

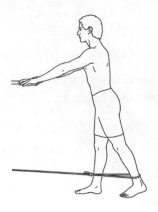

Chapter 2: Core Stability

Core stability refers to the ability of the lumbar spine and pelvis to support themselves in proper alignment when engaged in movements or positions that challenge static positioning. These exercises require multi-directional control of the lumbar spine, usually with some component of instability. In most cases, a device that is inherently less stable than solid flooring, such as a ball or roller, is involved. In many cases, unilateral or uneven loading is the source of instability. It may be that the actual position of the lumbar spine and pelvis is to be held steady, or to move only slightly. The main difference between the stabilization exercises and the control exercises is that there is some force acting against control. These exercises are progressed either by increasing duration, repetitions, and/or resistances.

Anterior — 17 exercises

Posterior — 11 exercises

Ball Roll: Basic

With forearms on ball and back straight, begin to roll forward, progressively tensing abdominals. Breathing out, roll back to start position.

Caution: Do not hyperextend low back.

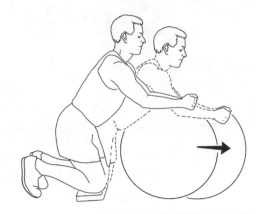

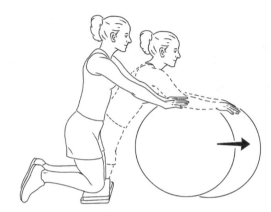

Ball Roll: Intermediate

With hands on ball and back straight, begin to roll forward, progressively tensing abdominals. Breathing out, roll back to start position.

Caution: Do not hyperextend low back.

Ball Roll: Advanced

With hands on ball, back straight, knees off the floor, begin to roll forward, progressively tensing abdominals. Breathing out, roll back to start position.

Caution: Do not hyperextend the low back.

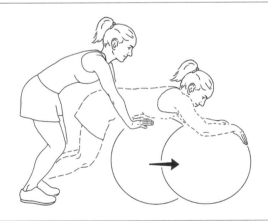

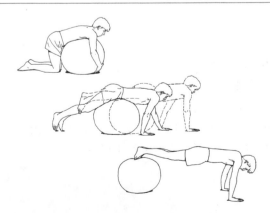

Kneeling Ball Walk to Thighs / Toes

Kneeling with stomach on ball, walk forward until it rests under thighs / toes.

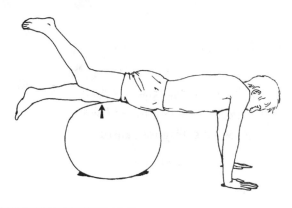

Prone Ball Walk to Thighs with Hip Extension

Walk forward on ball until it rests under thighs. Raise one thigh off ball. Repeat with other thigh.

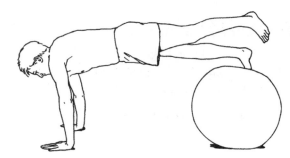

Prone Ball Walk to Toes with Hip Extension

Walk forward on ball until it rests under toes. Raise one leg off ball. Repeat with other leg.

Prone Ball Walk with Hip Abduction / Adduction

Walk forward on ball until it rests under thighs. Sweep one leg out to side and return. Repeat with other leg.

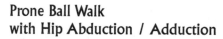
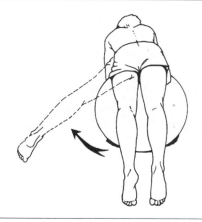

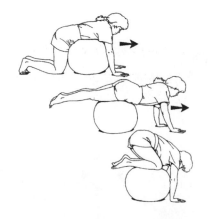

Kneeling Ball Walk to Double Knee to Chest

Walk forward on ball until it rests under shins. Support weight with hands and roll ball under you by bending knees up to chest.

Prone Ball Walk to "Skier" Position

With stomach on ball, walk forward until
ball rests under shins. Support weight
with hands and roll ball forward and
out to side by pulling with knees.

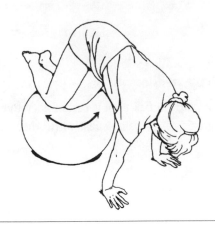

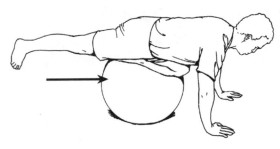

Prone Ball Walk to Single Knee to Chest

Walk forward on ball until it rests under
shins. Move one leg off ball and pull ball
leg to chest. Repeat with other leg.

Ball Roll (Supine)

Bridge trunk with head, neck, and shoulders
supported. Keeping arms extended and
parallel with shoulders, roll to one side
and hold. Repeat to other side.

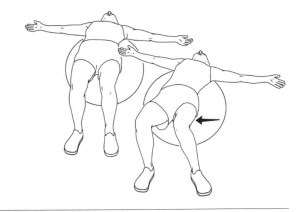

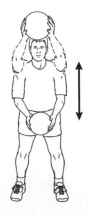

Front Chop

Hold a medicine ball with arms straight.
Rapidly move arms up and down.

Circle

Hold a medicine ball with arms straight. Rapidly move arms in circle counterclockwise, then counter clockwise.

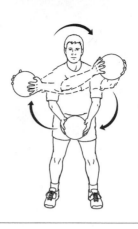

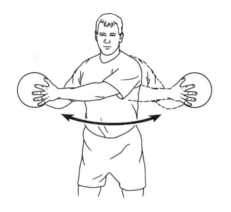

Rotational Chop

Hold a medicine ball with arms straight. Quickly rotate ball from side to side.

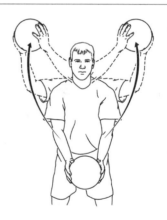

V Chop

Hold a medicine ball to chest. Quickly move arms in V shape: up and out, then down, then up and out on other side.

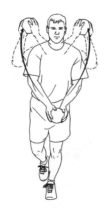

V Chop (Single Leg)

Balance on one leg, holding a medicine ball. Allowing elbows to bend, quickly move arms in V shape: up and out, then down, then up and out to other side.

Hip Chop

Hold a medicine ball at one hip. Quickly move ball from hip to above opposite shoulder and quickly return.

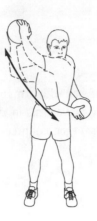

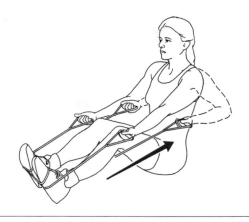

Low Row: Sitting

Tubing around feet and palms up, pull arms
back while squeezing shoulder blades together.

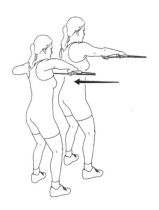

High Row: Standing

Face anchor, feet shoulder width
apart. Palms down, pull arms back,
squeezing shoulder blades together.

Low Row: Standing

Face anchor, feet shoulder width apart.
Palms up, pull arms back, squeezing
shoulder blades together.

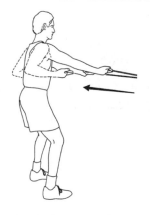

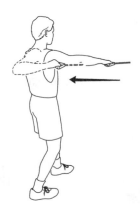

High Row: Single Arm

Face anchor in stride stance. Palm down, pull arm
back while squeezing shoulder blades together.

Low Row: Thumbs Up

Face anchor, medium to wide stance. Thumbs up, pull arms back, squeezing shoulder blades together.

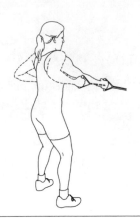

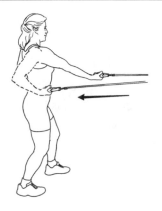

Low Row: Single Arm

Face anchor in stride stance. Palm up, pull arm back while squeezing shoulder blades together.

Low Row: Thumb Up (Single Arm)

Face anchor in stride stance. Thumb up, pull arm back, squeezing shoulder blades together.

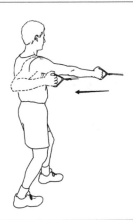

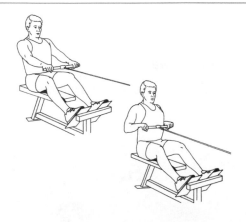

Row: Sitting (Cable)

Torso erect, pull bar to lower chest.

Row: Sitting – Wide Grip (Cable)

Torso erect, pull bar to chest.

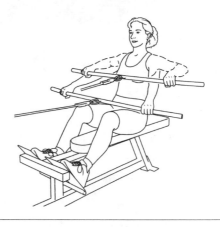

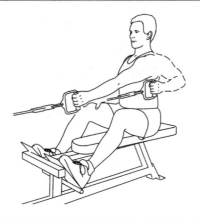

Row: Sitting – Single Arm (Cable)

Torso erect, bracing other hand on thigh, pull arm back to side of chest.

Row: Sitting (V-Bar, Cable)

Torso erect, pull bar to chest.

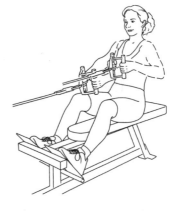

Chapter 3: Core Strength

Core strength exercises engage large groups of muscles performing large movements of the lumbar spine and pelvis. They are not subtle; rather, they involve forceful contractions of the prime movers making visible movements in a particular direction. These exercises may be calisthenic or include a piece of resistance equipment such as a free weight or machine. They may be more isolating, requiring less coordination than core control, stability, or function exercises. Strength exercises will be prescribed in much the same manner as for any other body part although most professionals tend to perform high repetitions with low resistances. Depending on one's fitness goals, progressions can be in duration, frequency, and/or intensity.

Anterior — 81 exercises

Posterior — 21 exercises

Crunch: Bent Knee

Arms straight, tighten abdominals, raise shoulders and upper back toward ceiling. Keep head and neck in line with spine. Keep low and middle back on floor.

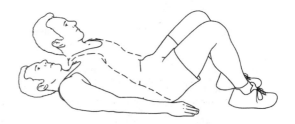

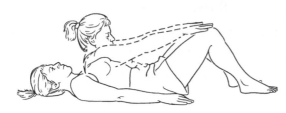

Curl-Up: Phase 1

With arms at sides, tilt pelvis to flatten back. Raise head and shoulders from floor. Use arms to support trunk if necessary. Hold.

The Hundred

Lie on back, straight legs slightly turned out. Inhale, reaching arms over head. Exhale, pressing arms down to sides, lift legs up to 45°, curling up head, upper torso. Hold. Keep low back pressed to mat. Pump arms in small flutters up and down.

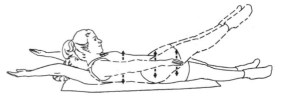

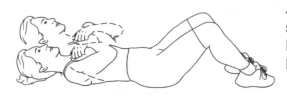

Crunch: Bent Knee

Arms crossed, tighten abdominals, raise shoulders and upper back toward ceiling. Keep head and neck in line with spine. Keep low and middle back on floor.

Crunch: Bent Knee

Arms behind head, tighten abdominals, raise shoulders and upper back toward ceiling. Keep head and neck in line with spine. Keep low and middle back on floor.

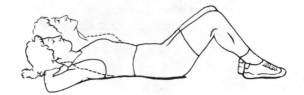

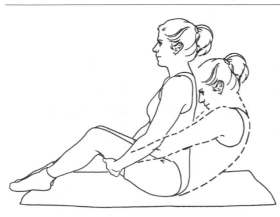

Half Roll-Down

Sit straight, legs bent, hands under thighs. Exhale, slowly rounding back halfway. Inhale, returning.

NOTE: Do not hunch shoulders.

Sit-Up: Bent Knee

Arms straight, tighten abdominals, bend at waist, curling upper body toward knees.

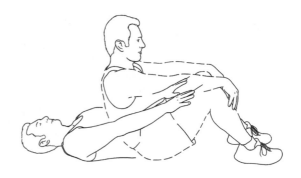

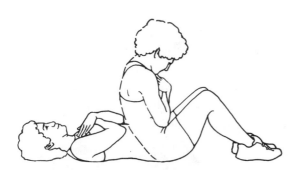

Sit-Up: Bent Knee

Arms crossed, tighten abdominals, bend at waist, curling upper body toward knees.

Sit-Up: Bent Knee

Hands at head, tighten abdominals, bend at waist, curling upper body toward knees.

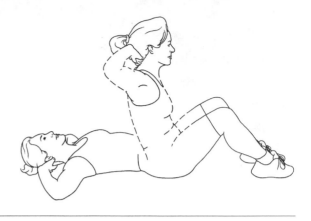

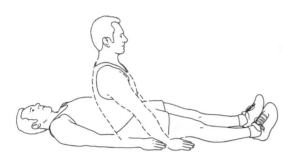

Sit-Up: Three-Quarter – Straight Leg

Arms straight, tighten abdominals, raise upper body three-quarters of the way to perpendicular with floor. Keep back straight.

Sit-Up: Three-Quarter – Straight Leg

Arms crossed, tighten abdominals, raise upper body three-quarters of the way to perpendicular with floor. Keep back straight.

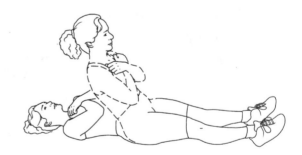

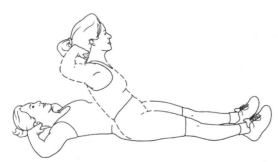

Sit-Up: Three-Quarter – Straight Leg

Hands at head, tighten abdominals, raise upper body three-quarters of the way to perpendicular with floor. Keep back straight.

Sit-Up: Medicine Ball at Chest

Cross arms on chest over medicine ball. Perform a sit-up.

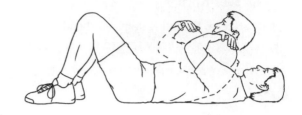

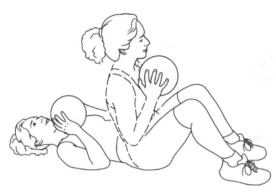

Sit-Up: Medicine Ball at Chest

Holding medicine ball to chest, sit up.

Sit-Up: Medicine Ball Over Head

Hold medicine ball beyond head. Perform a sit-up.

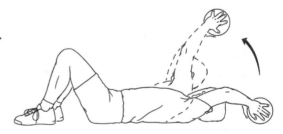

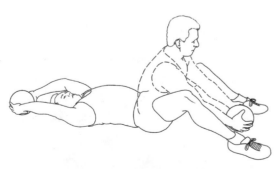

Sit-Up: Medicine Ball Over Head

Holding medicine ball beyond head, sit up, touching ball to floor between feet.

Catch (Medicine Ball)

Interlock legs. Tighten abdominals and alternate sit-up motions with partner while gently tossing a medicine ball to each other.

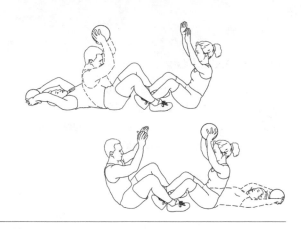

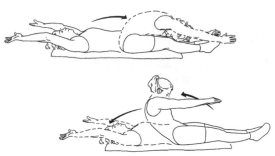

Roll-Up (Intermediate / Advanced)

Lie on back, straight legs together, slightly turned out, arms over head. Exhale, rolling up spine, arms reaching forward over legs. Inhale, rolling back halfway. Exhale, rolling down to start.

NOTE: Do not hunch shoulders.

Partial Sit-Up: Lower Abdominals

With legs over footstool or chair, and arms clasped behind neck or folded across chest, tilt pelvis to flatten back. Raise head and shoulders from floor.

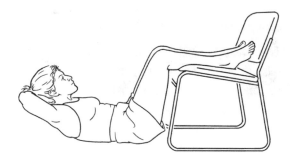

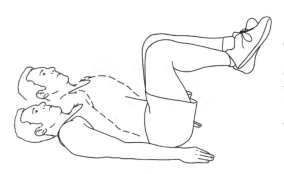

Crunch: Raised Leg

Arms straight, legs up, bent, ankles crossed, tighten abdominals, raise shoulders and upper back toward ceiling. Keep head and neck in line with spine. Keep low and middle back on floor.

Crunch: Raised Leg

Arms crossed, legs up, bent, ankles crossed, tighten abdominals, raise shoulders and upper back toward ceiling. Keep head and neck in line with spine. Keep low and middle back on floor.

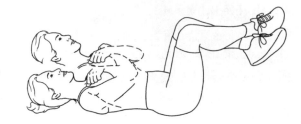

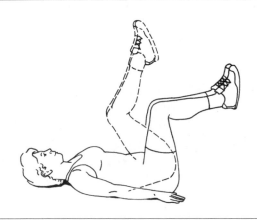

Crunch: Reverse

With knees at 90° angle, tighten abdominals, curl hips up until low back clears floor.

Sit-Up: Jack Knife

Tighten abdominals, simultaneously raise upper body and legs, attempting to touch hands to feet or ankles.

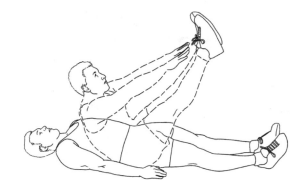

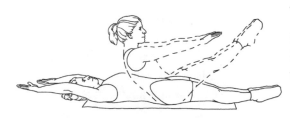

Teaser

Lie on back, arms over head. Exhale, rising to balance on seat in V position. Inhale at top, then exhale, slowly rolling down to start.

Sit-Up: Jack Knife – Alternating

Tighten abdominals, simultaneously raise upper body and one leg, attempting to touch hands to foot or ankle. Alternate legs.

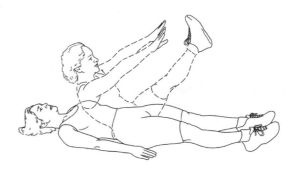

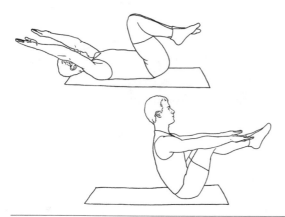

Teaser I

Lie on back, knees to chest, arms over head. Exhale, curling up to sitting, balanced on seat, legs bent 90°. Inhale at top, then exhale, slowly rolling down to start.

Crunch: Decline

Tighten abdominals, raise shoulders and upper back toward ceiling. Keep head and neck in line with spine. Keep low and middle back on bench.

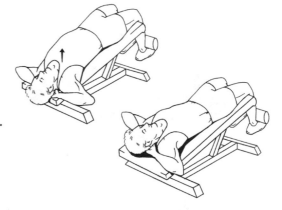

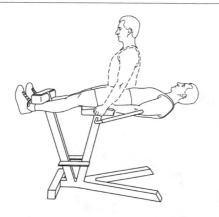

Sit-Up (Roman Chair)

Upper body parallel to floor, tighten abdominals, sit up.

Sit-Up: Full Range (Roman Chair)

Body bent toward floor in comfortable
position, tighten abdominals, sit up.

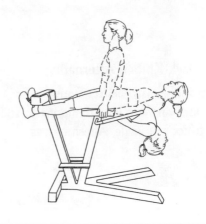

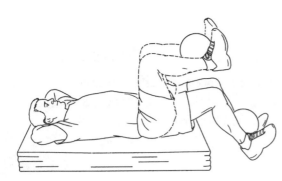

Reverse Curl (Supine)

Lie on back, holding medicine ball between
feet, knees bent 90°. Lift knees toward chest.

Reverse Curl / Crunch (Supine)

Lie on back, holding medicine ball between
feet, knees bent 90°. Lift knees toward
chest while lifting upper body.

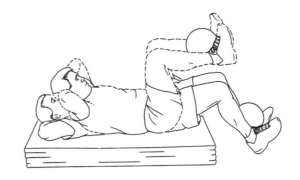

Leg Lift (Supine)

Lie on back, holding medicine ball between
feet. Lift legs and ball off floor.

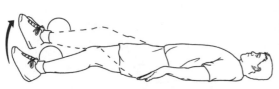

Knee Raise (Sitting)

Tighten abdominals and bend legs, pulling knees toward chest.

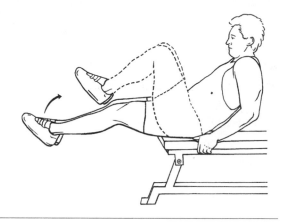

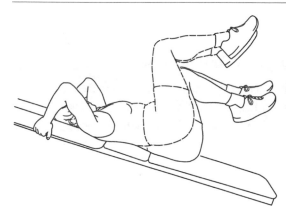

Caudal Flexion: Knee Lift – Incline

Lie holding support, knees together and up, bent to 90°. Curl lower abdominals, lifting knees and hips toward ceiling, keeping legs at 90°.

Reverse Curl (V Sitting on Mat)

Sit on mat, holding medicine ball between feet, knees straight. Lean back from hips and hold. Lift knees toward chest.

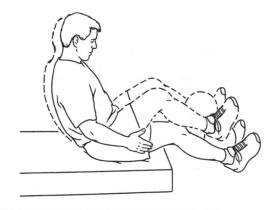

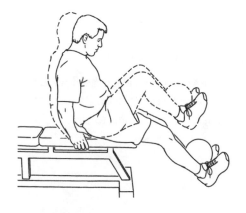

Reverse Curl (V Sitting on Bench)

Sit on bench, holding medicine ball between feet, knees straight. Lean back from hips and hold. Lift knees toward chest.

Saw

Sit up straight, legs open slightly wider than hips. Extend arms to side, flex feet. Inhale, twisting to side. Exhale, rounding spine over leg, reach opposite hand toward outside of foot, other arm back, palm up.

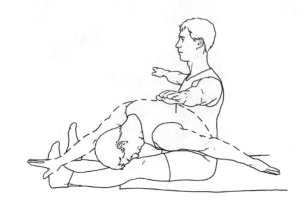

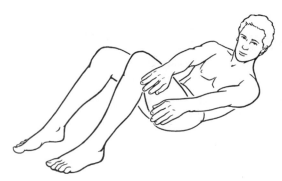

Diagonal Curl-Up: Phase 1

With arms at sides, tilt pelvis to flatten back. Raise head and shoulders, rotating to side as shoulder blades clear floor. Hold.

Diagonal Curl-Up: Phase 2

Keeping arms folded across chest, tilt pelvis to flatten back. Lift head and shoulders from floor while rotating to side. Hold.

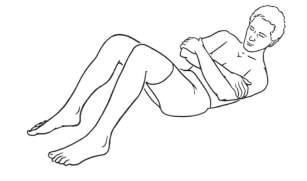

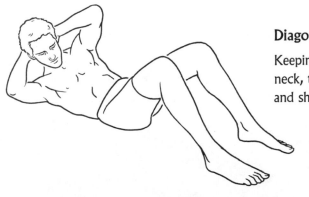

Diagonal Curl-Up: Phase 3

Keeping hands clasped behind head to support neck, tilt pelvis to flatten back. Raise head and shoulders while rotating to side. Hold.

Crunch: Twist – Bent Leg

One ankle across other knee, tighten abdominals, twist upper body to touch opposite elbow to knee. Do all repetitions to one side. Repeat to other side.

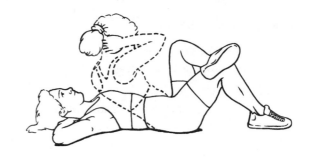

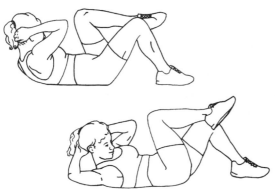

Crunch: Twist – Bent Leg, Alternating

Legs bent, tighten abdominals, raise upper body and one leg. Twist to touch opposite elbow to raised knee. Alternate sides.

Crisscross

Lie on back, legs bent to chest, hands behind head. Exhale, lifting head and upper torso. Twist torso and elbow to opposite knee. Inhale, twisting to other side.

NOTE: Keep navel to spine, back flat.

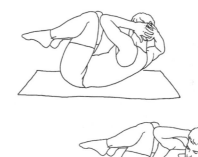

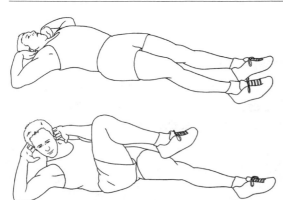

Crunch: Scissor Kick / Twist

Tighten abdominals, raise upper body, twist to side, and touch elbow to opposite raised knee. Alternate sides.

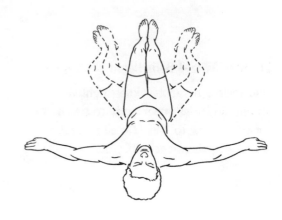

Lower Trunk Rotation

Bring both knees in to chest. Rotate from side to side, keeping knees together and feet off floor. Hold each position.

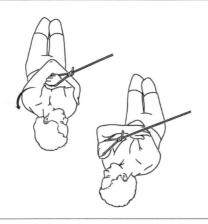

Lumbar Rotation: Resisted (Supine)

With side toward anchor, without moving pelvis, rotate upper body away from anchor in a pain-free range of motion.

Sit-Up: Twist – Bent Knee

Tighten abdominals, twist upper body, touching elbow to inside of opposite knee. Alternate sides.

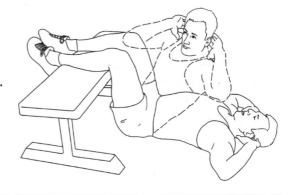

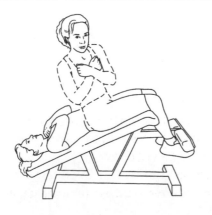

Sit-Up: Twist – Decline

Arms crossed on chest, tighten abdominals, raise upper body, twisting to side. Keep back straight. Alternate sides.

Lumbar Rotation: Resisted (Sitting)

Feet toward anchor, tubing looped around upper left arm, rotate trunk.

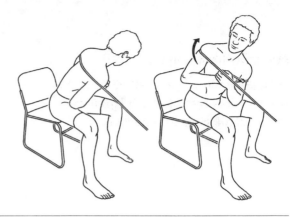

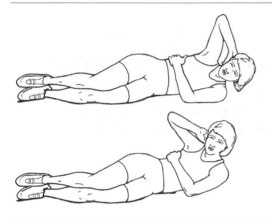

Crunch: Side

With knees bent, tighten abdominals, flex upper body upward, moving elbow toward hip.

Side Bend: Caudal (Side-Lying)

Lying on hip and elbow, lift pelvis, keeping elbow and feet on board.

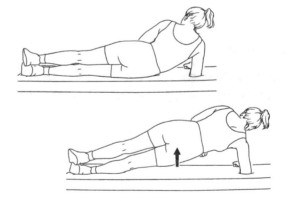

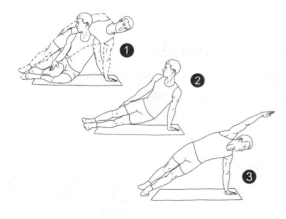

Side Bend

Sit on side of hip, knees bent, hand on mat, other arm on side.

1. Inhale, pressing up to straight line.
2. Exhale, lowering hips halfway, turning head to side.
3. Inhale, pressing up straight, extending arm beyond head. Exhale, returning to sit.

Hip Lift: Side-Lying (Gymball)

Lie on side with feet together on ball. Support head with hand. Lift hips in line with knees. Repeat on other side.

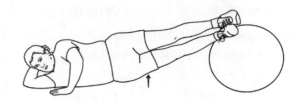

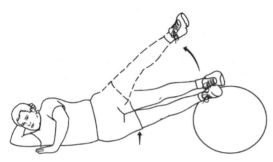

Hip Lift with Leg Lift: Side-Lying (Gymball)

Lie on side with feet together on ball. Support head with hand. Lift hips then lift top leg. Repeat on other side.

Side Bend (Dumbbell)

Tighten abdominals and bend to side as far as possible.

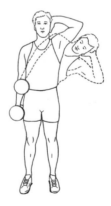

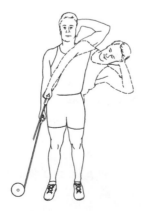

Side Bend (Cable)

Tighten abdominals and bend to side as far as possible. Complete all repetitions to one side. Repeat to other side.

Side Bend: Cranial Trunk (Incline Board)

Lie on side on incline board with bolster under hip. Hands clasped behind head, tighten stomach and lift shoulders.

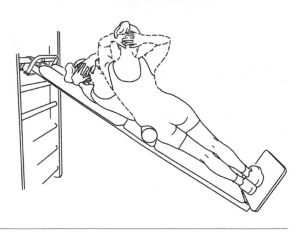

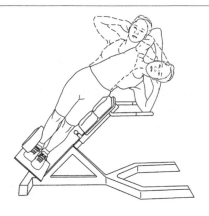

Hyperextension: Side

Body bent at waist to side, tighten abdominals, bring upper body up, in line with legs.

Hyperextension: Side – Partner Assist

Partner stabilizes legs. Upper body bent at waist toward floor, tighten abdominals, flex upward as far as possible.

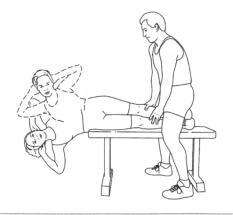

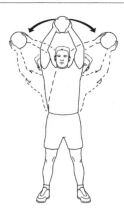

Lateral Bend (Standing)

Hold medicine ball over head. Bend to one side, then the other.

Abdominal Curl: Kneeling

Face away from anchor, kneeling. Hands overlapping behind neck, curl forward.

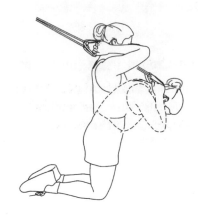

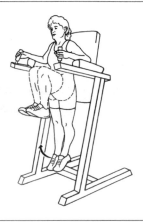

Knee Raise

Tighten abdominals and bending legs, pulling knees toward chest.

Knee Raise: Hanging

Tighten abdominals and bending legs, pulling knees toward chest.

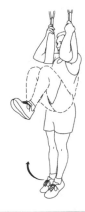

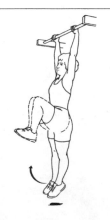

Knee Raise: Hanging

Tighten abdominals and bending legs, pulling knees toward chest.

Abdominal Wheel

Tighten abdominals and roll out without allowing upper body or arms to touch ground. Return to starting position.

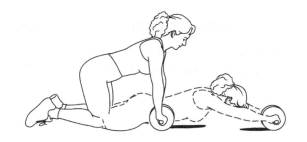

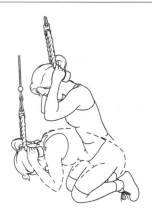

Crunch: Cable

Tighten abdominals and curl upper body downward moving elbows toward knees.

Crunch: Sitting (Machine)

Chest against pad, tighten abdominals and curl upper body toward knees.

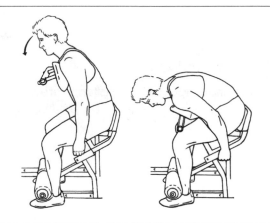

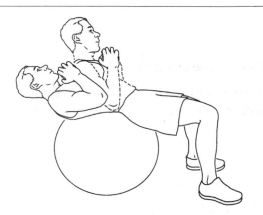

Crunch (Dumbbell)

Hold dumbbell on upper chest, low back supported. Tighten abdominals by bringing ribs toward pelvis until shoulders clear ball.

Crunch: Alternating (Dumbbell)

Hold dumbbell on upper chest, low back supported. Tighten abdominals by bringing right ribs toward left pelvis. Repeat to other side.

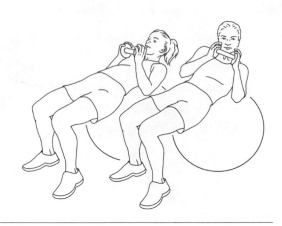

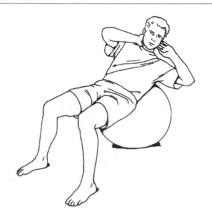

Diagonal Curl-Up: Supine on Ball

From reclined position, perform diagonal curl-up, bringing one elbow toward opposite knee. Repeat to other side.

Half Sit-Up: Sitting

From incline sitting position, perform curl-up.

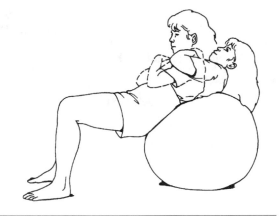

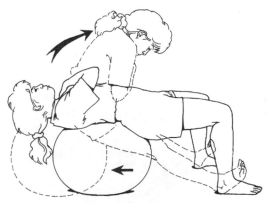

Full Sit-Up: Sitting

From reclined position, perform sit-up. End with body perpendicular to straightened legs.

Crunch (Cable)

Grasp rope handle, low back supported. Tighten abdominals by bringing ribs toward pelvis until shoulders clear ball.

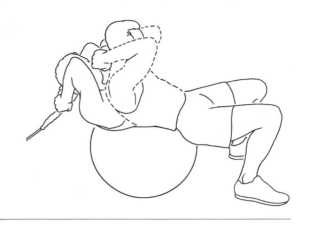

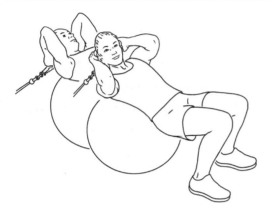

Crunch: Alternating (Cable)

Grasp rope handle, low back supported. Tighten abdominals by bringing one side of ribs toward opposite side of pelvis until shoulder clears ball. Repeat to other side.

Crunch: Seated (Cable)

Grasp rope handle over head. Tighten abdominals by bringing elbows toward knees. Only spine moves.

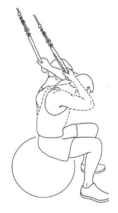

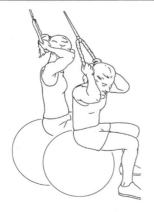

Crunch: Seated – Alternating (Cable)

Grasp rope handle over head. Tighten abdominals by bringing elbow toward opposite knee. Repeat to other side. Only spine moves.

Crunch: Reverse – Alternating

Grasp a stable bar, legs bent, hips at 90°.
Keeping abdominals tensed, extend hips
then reverse direction by bringing knees
toward shoulder. Repeat to other side.

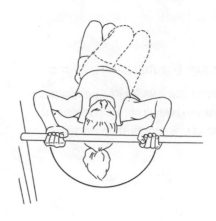

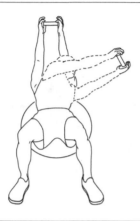

Twist: Supine (Dumbbell)

Bridge trunk, head, neck and shoulders
supported, arms extended over head holding
dumbbell. Rotate trunk to side, keeping
arms extended. Repeat to other side.

Crunch: Reverse

Grasp a stable bar, legs bent, hips
at 90°. Keeping abdominals tensed,
extend hips then reverse direction.

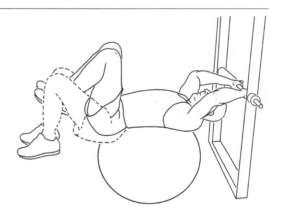

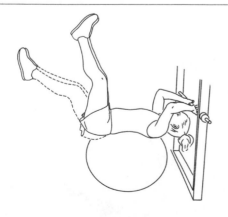

Straight Leg Raise

Grasp stable bar. Keeping abdominals tensed,
extend hips then reverse direction.

Straight Leg Raise: Alternating

Grasp stable bar. Keeping abdominals tensed, extend one hip then reverse direction. Repeat with other leg.

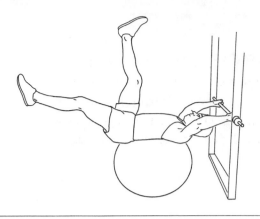

Bridging

Slowly raise buttocks from floor,
keeping stomach tight. Hold.

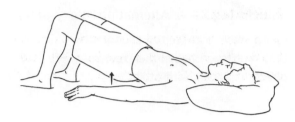

Arm / Leg Lift: Opposite (Prone)

Lift one leg and opposite arm from
floor, keeping knee locked. Hold.

Upper Body Extension

With support under abdomen, clasp hands
behind back and lift upper body from floor.
Keep chin tucked while lifting. Hold.

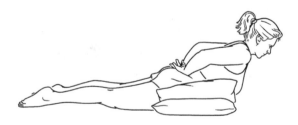

Back Extension (Prone)

With support under abdomen, lift upper body
and legs from floor. Do not arch neck. Hold.

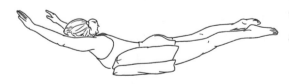

Back Extension / Rotation: Cranial (Prone)

With support under abdomen and hips, one hand behind head, other hand behind back. Lift head and trunk, rotating top elbow up and back.

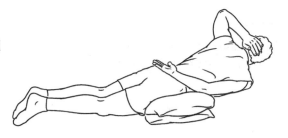

Trunk Extension (Prone)

Lie prone, holding medicine ball out in front. Lift chest and ball off floor.

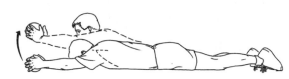

Trunk Extension / Rotation (Prone)

Lie prone, holding medicine ball out in front. Lift and rotate upper body to one side and then the other, ball off floor.

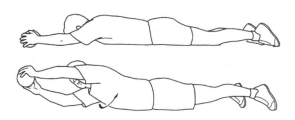

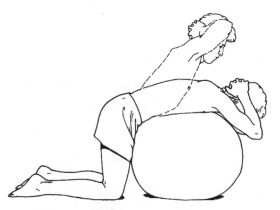

Back Extension (Kneeling)

With hands on back of head, extend upper back from ball.

Back Extension (Prone)

With hands on back of head,
lift upper back from ball.

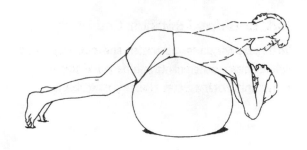

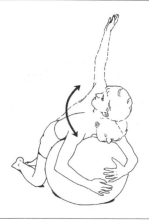

One Arm Raise with Spinal Rotation (Prone, Kneeling)

From kneeling, raise one arm while rotating
trunk into position shown. Hold.

Segmental Flexion / Extension

Clasp hands behind head and slowly bend
down, segment by segment, through lower
back. To return, first raise chin, then
straighten neck, upper back, and so on.

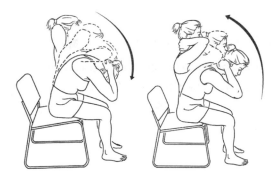

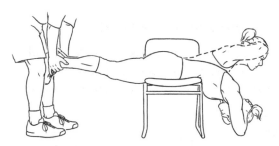

Upper Back Extension: Partner (Over Chair)

On stomach over chair, partner
anchoring feet, raise torso, keeping
hands behind neck for support.

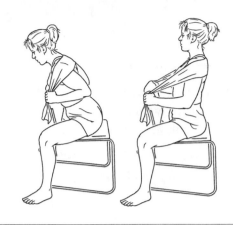

Back Extension: Resisted

Sitting backward in chair with resistive band held against chair back and looped around upper body, lean back against resistance of band.

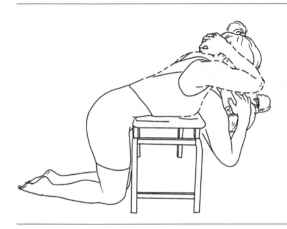

Back Extension: Cranial Segmental – Trunk Support (Prone Kneeling)

Bend over bench, then reach elbows forward and up, extending spine from head to low back, one segment at a time.

Back Extension (Kneeling)

Buttocks toward heels and upper body forward, raise head, chest, and arms.

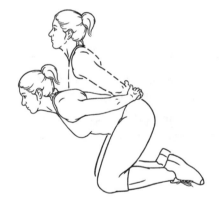

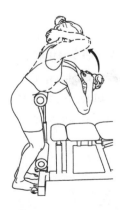

Back Extension: Segmental (Block)

Knees against support, bend forward over roll. Reach elbows forward and up, extending spine from head to low back, one segment at a time.

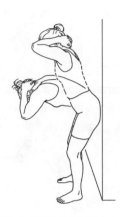

Back Extension: Cranial Segmental

Seat against wall, bend forward. Reach elbows forward and up, extending spine from head to low back, one segment at a time.

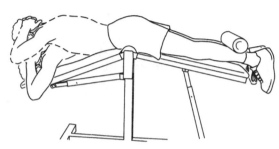

Back Extension: Cranial – Prone (Foot Fixation)

Clasp hands behind head. Extend spine by lifting head and shoulders off bench.

Caution: Do not hyperextend.

Low Back Extension

Bent at hips, back straight, hands behind head, raise torso until in line with legs.

Caution: Do NOT extend past parallel to floor.

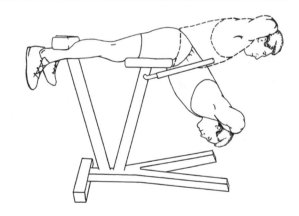

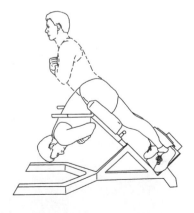

Low Back Extension: Incline

Bent at hips, back straight, hands crossed on chest, raise torso until in line with legs.

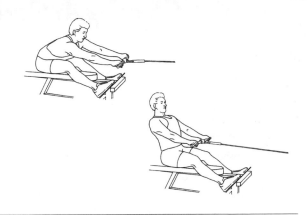

Row: Stiff Arm

Stretched forward, straighten back until
slightly past perpendicular to floor.

Chapter 4: Core Function

Exercises for core function are those which simulate real-world movements and actions. They most likely require anterior and posterior muscles to work together, often with pelvic muscles. They tend to occur in positions that are vertical, such as sitting or standing, and consist of movements that are dynamic. Advanced trainees may even use some of these movements ballistically or plyometrically. They usually include a resistance tool such as a medicine ball or tubing. It is recommended that a foundation of core control, stability, and strength be established prior to implementing these exercises. Proper form is essential both for movement transfer as well as spinal safety. Finally, core function exercises are often progressed in numbers of repetitions, sets, or speed and should be terminated at the first sign of technical breakdown, not total fatigue.

Anterior — 21 exercises

Posterior — 22 exercises

Trunk Rotation: Sitting (Tubing)

Sitting, side to anchor, hold tubing with arms across chest. Rotate trunk away.

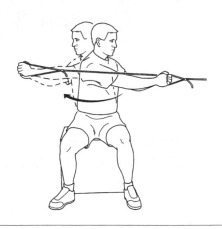

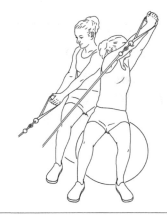

Wood Chop: Sitting (Cable)

Grasp cable and rotate trunk by bringing hands toward opposite hip. Keep pelvis stable.

Wood Chop: Reverse – Sitting (Cable)

Grasp cable and rotate trunk by bringing hands above opposite shoulder. Keep pelvis stable.

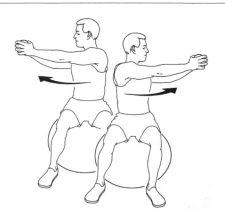

Trunk Rotation: Sitting (Dumbbell)

Grasp dumbbell with arms horizontal. Rotate trunk by bringing arms across body. Keep pelvis stable.

Trunk Rotation: Kneeling (Tubing)

Kneeling, side toward anchor, hold tubing with arms across chest. Rotate trunk away.

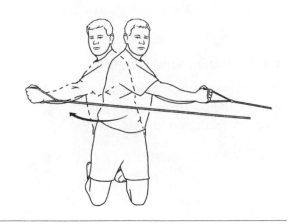

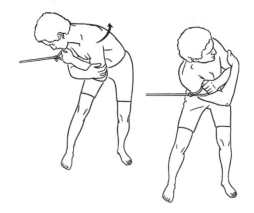

Lumbar Rotation: Resisted – Standing

Side toward anchor, with knees slightly bent and back straight, bend forward at hips. Maintaining posture, rotate away from anchor in a pain-free range of motion.

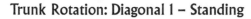

Trunk Rotation: Diagonal 1 – Standing

Lean forward toward anchor in shoulder width stance. Tubing around anchor-side hand, hold at opposite shoulder. Rotate trunk up and away from anchor.

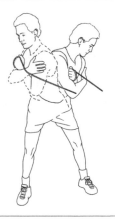

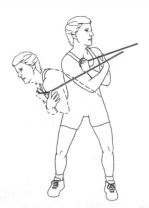

Trunk Rotation: Diagonal 2 – Standing

Side toward anchor in shoulder width stance. Turn upper body toward anchor. Tubing around anchor-side hand, hold at opposite shoulder. Rotate trunk down and away from anchor.

Trunk Twist: Standing

Side toward anchor in wide stance, reach toward anchor. Thumbs up, pull away from anchor. Keep arm furthest from anchor straight.

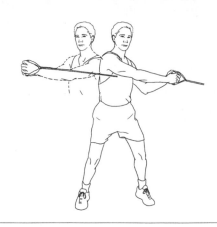

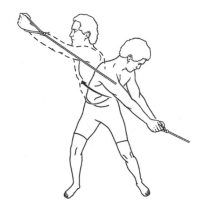

Lumbar Diagonal Rotation #2: Resisted - Standing

Side toward anchor, feet slightly offset, reach down across body. Straighten upper body, rotating up to other side.

Lumbar Diagonal Rotation #1: Resisted - Standing

Side toward anchor, reach up and out to same side. Bend body, rotating down to other side.

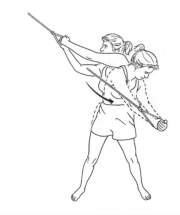

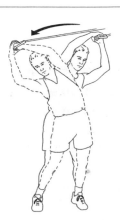

Trunk Side Bend: Standing

Side toward anchor in wide stance, arms above head, tilt trunk toward anchor. Grasp handle and pull away from anchor.

Trunk Flexion (Tubing)

Hold tubing anchored high on each side, arms stretched over head, palms forward. Pull hands down to outside of opposite foot, palms back.

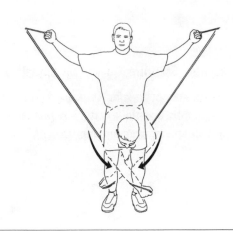

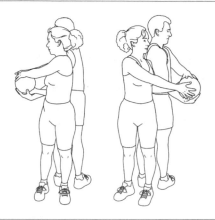

Pass (Medicine Ball)

Stand back-to-back. Tighten abdominals and twist at waist, passing ball, alternating sides. Keep lower body stationary.

Diagonal: Standing

Clasp hands together over head holding dumbbells. Reach down to outside of one foot. Raise arms over head to opposite side. Repeat to other foot for set.

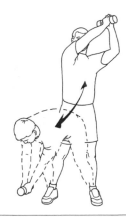

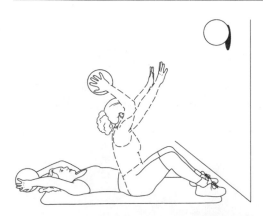

Sit-Up: Wall Throw (Medicine Ball)

Holding medicine ball beyond head, sit up and bounce ball off wall.

Wall Tap: Over Head (Medicine Ball)

Stand close to wall. Envision a clock face on wall. Using small motions at the hip and trunk, tap ball against wall each "hour", 10 - 2.

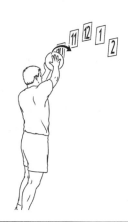

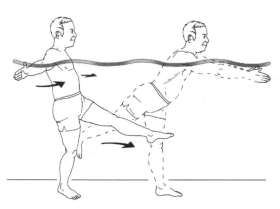

Rocking Horse (Aquatic)

Stand, arms out from sides, one leg raised forward. Push from back leg onto front leg, as arms move forward and together. Then push from front leg onto back leg, as arms move apart.

Straight Leg Lift (Aquatic)

Move one leg forward and up, knee straight. Reach with opposite arm toward toes while bringing other arm out behind.

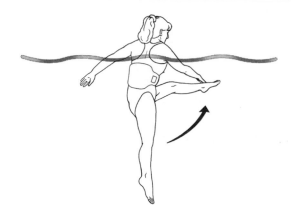

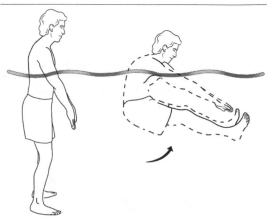

Kick Forward Jump (Aquatic)

Stand with legs apart, arms forward. Bend trunk and kick legs up toward hands with a jump.

Trunk Lateral Flexion: Pendulum (Aquatic)

Swing both legs from one side to other, keeping knees straight and together. Movement should come from hips and trunk.

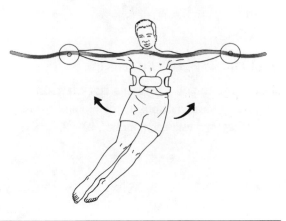

Dead Lift (Barbell)

From squat, straighten legs, keeping head up and back straight.

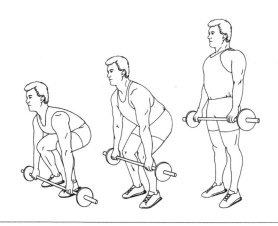

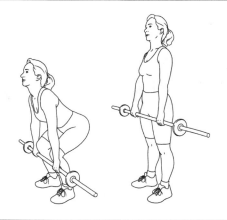

Dead Lift: Three Quarter (Barbell)

From three quarter squat position, straighten legs, keeping head up and back straight.

Dead Lift (Dumbbell)

Legs straight, back flat, raise torso until in line with legs.

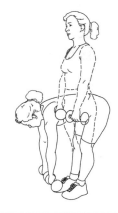

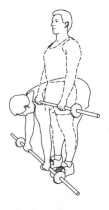

Dead Lift: Straight-Leg (Barbell)

Legs straight, back flat, raise torso until in line with legs.

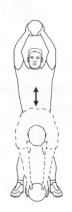

Trunk Flexion / Extension (Standing)

Hold medicine ball over head. Touch ball to floor, bending knees as necessary.

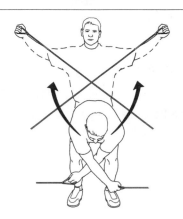

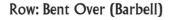

Trunk Extension (Tubing)

Arms crossed, hold tubing anchored low on each side, hands outside of feet, palms back. Straighten trunk, reaching up and out, palms forward.

Row: Bent Over (Barbell)

Lift barbell to chest, keeping back flat and knees bent.

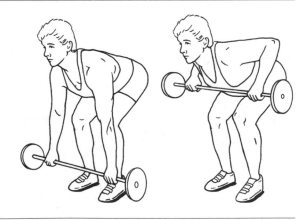

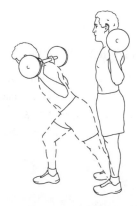

Back Extension: Anterior Fall-Out Lunge

Step forward on one leg, keeping front knee over ankle, back straight, heel on floor. Keep trunk in line with back leg. Push off front leg to return. Alternate legs.

Pull Simulation: Resisted

Face anchor, reach forward. Keeping arms straight, lean back.

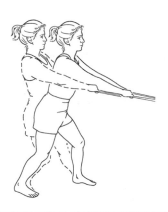

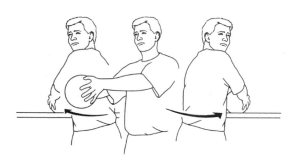

Trunk Rotation

Stand with back to counter top. Hold medicine ball. Turn and place ball on counter. Twist to opposite side and pick up ball. Turn and place ball on counter.

Partner Drill: Rotational Pass – Two-Handed

Holding medicine ball, stand away from partner. Rotate away and back, tossing ball. Partner catches ball and does same.

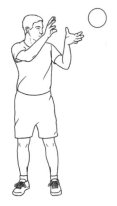

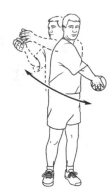

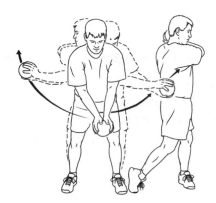

Golf Swing (One Ball)

Holding medicine ball in both hands at address, perform full golf swing, reaching as far as possible both directions.

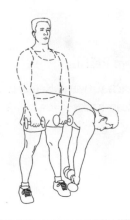

Dead Lift: Twisting (Dumbbell)

Legs straight, back flat, torso twisted, hold dumbbells at outside of one foot. Bring body up, twisting to forward. Alternate sides.

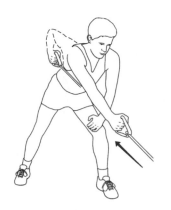

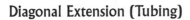

Low Row: Bent Over – Thumb Up, Single Arm

Face anchor in wide stride stance. Thumb up, pull arm back, squeezing shoulder blades together.

Diagonal Extension (Tubing)

Side toward low anchor, hold tubing with both hands outside foot. Pull up and across, reaching over opposite shoulder.

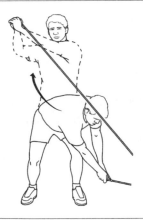

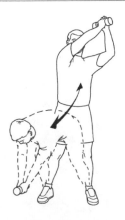

Diagonal: Chop (Standing)

Clasp hands together over head holding dumbbell. Reach down to outside of one foot. Raise arms over head to opposite side. Repeat to other foot for set.

Golf Swing (Two Balls)

Holding medicine ball in hands and one between arms, perform full golf swing, reaching as far as possible both directions.

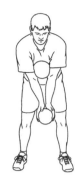
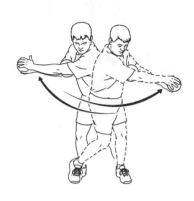

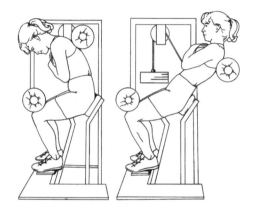

Low Back Extension (Machine)

Torso forward, back straight, extend torso backward, until it aligns with hips.

Good Morning (Barbell)

Bent 90° at hips, knees slightly bent, head up, back straight, raise torso until in line with legs.

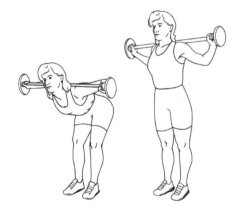

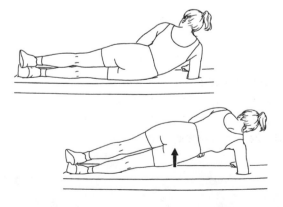

Side-Bend: Caudal – Side-Lying

Lying on hip and elbow, lift pelvis, keeping elbow and feet on board.

Hip Lift: Side-Lying (Gymball)

Lie on side with feet together on ball. Support head with hand. Lift hips in line with knees.

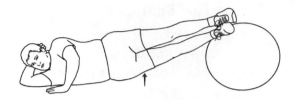

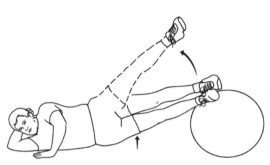

Hip Lift with Leg Lift: Side-Lying (Gymball)

Lie on side with feet together on ball. Support head with hand. Lift hips then lift top leg.

About VHI

Visual Health Information (VHI) is the leading publisher of reproducible exercise tools. VHI has been producing exercise collections for the rehabilitation and fitness markets since 1980.

VHI produces reproducible exercise cards and computer software. VHI has over 35 different exercise collections. These collections include exercises for Outpatient Physical Therapy, Geriatrics, Pediatrics, Fitness, Strength & Conditioning, Pre/Postnatal, Speech, Pulmonary Rehab and much more.

The content for the Exercise Idea book series is derived from the over 9,000 exercise images in the VHI exercise database. These books are designed to show you the wide range of exercises that can be used for specific purposes.

To view all the VHI offerings and collections, visit **www.vhikits.com,** or call **1-800-356-0709.**